Food or Poison

Revealing the Truth about What You Eat and Its Impact on Your Well-Being

TOBY BRYANT

ACKNOWLEDGMENT 5

COPYRIGHT 5

FORWARD 6

Moving forward 6

CHAPTER 1 8

Importance Of Diet in Overall Health and Well-Being. 8

The Impact of Diet on Our Lives 9

Beyond Physical Health: The Impact on Mood and Mind 11

A Quiet Supporter Against Illness 12

The Quest for Longevity 13

CHAPTER 2 18

The Basics of Nutrition 18

Why is eating well important? 19

CHAPTER 3 24

The Modern Diet Dilemma 24

The Varied Spectrum of Diets 27

The Processed Food Pitfalls 29

CHAPTER 4 32

Food and diseases: What to know to ensure food safety 32

Heart Disease 33

DIABETES 36

OBESITY 39

CHAPTER 5 43

Food as Medicine 43

The Healing Power of Food: Nourishing the Body, Mind, and Soul 43

Foods with Functions: Not Just Nutrition 49

Using Food as Medicine in Everyday Living 51

CHAPTER 6 56

Exposing Diet Myths: Dispelling 20 Common Misconceptions. 56

20 Common Myth about Diet 56

CHAPTER 7 64

Mindful Eating and Portion Control 64

The Deep Dive into the Art of Mindful Eating 64

Achievable Techniques for Mindful Consumption and Portion Management: 68

Creating Well-Balanced Meals: A Culinary Journey: 70

CHAPTER 8 76

Customized Nutrition: Creating a Diet That Is Unique to You 76

The Personalized Nutrition Foundations 76

Putting Personalized Nutrition into Practice 78

Practical Applications of Personalized Nutrition 79

The Future of Nutrition: Empowering Individuals 80

The Practical and Ethical Aspects of Tailored Nutrition 81

Putting Customized Nutrition into Practice: A Step Towards Holistic Health 82

CHAPTER 9 84

Selecting Sustainable Foods 84

Sustainable Eating: What Is It? 84

Food's Environmental Footprint 86

How to Choose Sustainable Foods 88

CHAPTER 10 92

Implementing Positive Changes 92

Final Thoughts: A Path of Self-Care and Nourishing 96

CHAPTER 11 97

Recipes and Meal Plans 97

SAMPLE MEAL PLAN 100

CHAPTER 12 108

The Journey Ahead 108

ACKNOWLEDGMENT

I would like to extend my heartfelt gratitude to all those who contributed to the creation of this book, "Food or Poison: It is Love at first sight for this undertaking that is a labor of love and a shared vision towards a healthier and more mindful world. Therefore, I would like to thank my relatives and companions who always stood beside me during the whole period of study. I need to say that your faith in our project and your readiness to help are very significant to me.

To the readers that may read out on this and those making a change. This book was written especially for you, and I hope it will be of useful assistance in your journey towards wellness.

Last but not least, I want to thank all the researchers, nutritionists, and health specialists whose research made it possible to have access to this deep understanding of the relationship between nutrition and health. It was a never-ending inspiration for me that you devoted your whole life to the nutrition area.

Appreciation to everyone who participated in the process. Let us build a healthier and more mindful future for all of us together.

COPYRIGHT

FORWARD

Moving forward

"Food or Poison: Revealing the Truth about What You Eat and Its Impact on Your Well-Being" is a helpful guide through the sometimes-confusing world of nutrition in a world where advice about what to eat and what to avoid is a common occurrence. This book is an invitation to go out on a path toward a more thoughtful, healthful relationship with food rather than just a compilation of statistics and data. You will discover an investigation of the deep relationship between the nourishment we take in and the life we lead as we turn the pages of this book. We solve the riddles of macronutrients and micronutrients and their crucial roles in our well-being as we explore the science underlying the nutrients that power our bodies, from the macro to the micro.

As we analyze typical dietary patterns, get ready to fight myths and dispel preconceived notions. "Food or Poison" offers a fair and fact-based viewpoint in a world where opinions often seem to veer to one side or the other, giving you the power to choose wisely what to put on your plate.

This book is a travel companion, not merely a repository of knowledge, with its helpful advice, delectable recipes, and individualized counsel. With an open mind, we ask you to turn the pages and be prepared to take in the wisdom and apply it to your own life.

Always keep in mind that the food decisions we make affect more than just our taste senses; they also nourish our bodies, fuel our aspirations, and, in the end, help shape our destiny.

CHAPTER 1
Importance Of Diet in Overall Health and Well-Being.

With everything going on in today's world, it might be easy to forget how much our decisions at the dinner table affect our overall health. But remember that there's much more to what you put on your plate than just convenience or flavor. It's a choice that will affect every aspect of your life, influencing your longevity, vitality, and even the standard of your days.

Take a moment to appreciate the human body's astounding complexity—a marvel of natural engineering. A symphony of biological processes controls every idea that enters your head and every beat of your heart. Your food is the foundation of this symphony; it provides the building blocks from which your body creates its masterwork.

The things you choose to eat are the building blocks of life itself, not just sources of nutrition. The fundamental components that provide your body with the energy and nourishment it needs for growth, repair, and peak performance are proteins, carbs, fats, vitamins, and minerals.

But that's not where the narrative ends. Your food is an important factor in determining your mental and emotional health as well as a quiet ally in your body's fight against disease and aging. Food affects your mood, cognitive performance, and even your capacity to handle stress. Its effects go well beyond the physical.

You will go on a voyage of exploration as we turn the pages of this book. Together, we will explore the science underlying the foods we eat and piece together the complex picture of nutrition. We will dispel myths and provide you with up-to-date research information, enabling you to make educated eating decisions.

Thus, approach this investigation of "food or poison" with an open mind and an inquiring heart. Acknowledge the possibility of change that every meal offers. Accept the ability you possess to mold, one mouthful at a time, a future of robust health and bright well-being.

The Impact of Diet on Our Lives

Let's begin by recognizing the significant influence that our food choices have on our quality of life. Food is frequently seen as just fuel in today's fast-paced world, something to be consumed while on the go. We seldom ever stop to think about how our dietary habits will affect us down the road.

Our bodies are amazing, complex machines. Numerous metabolic processes occur every second to maintain our health and survival. Our bodies are constantly working, whether it be with digestion or energy production. And the main fuel for this biological apparatus is the food we eat.

Think of it this way: The food you eat is the raw material, and your body is the construction site. Your body employs proteins, carbs, lipids, vitamins, and minerals as building blocks and tools to repair and sustain itself. The strength and longevity of the construction are directly impacted by the caliber of these materials.

Your mental and emotional well-being, in addition to your physical health, are significantly impacted by the things you put into your body. The correct nutrients work diligently to maintain your body in optimal operating order, much like trained artisans. Conversely, the incorrect ones might be compared to saboteurs, compromising your body's structural integrity and resulting in a host of health problems.

Beyond Physical Health: The Impact on Mood and Mind

Our food decisions have an impact on much more than just our physical well-being. Our emotional and mental health are closely linked to them. In addition to providing energy, food is a source of neurotransmitters, which are chemical messengers in our brains that convey impulses.

Think about this: Ever notice how a sugary treat may quickly boost your mood and give you energy, but then there's a crash that makes you feel tired and agitated? That is how food affects the chemistry of your brain.

Our diets have a significant impact on how our mood and brain activity are regulated. For instance, whole grains and other complex carbs give the brain a consistent flow of glucose, which supports a stable mood and maximum cognitive function. However, consuming too many processed sugars can cause blood sugar levels to fluctuate, which can exacerbate mood swings and cognitive fog.

Additionally, some nutrients—like the omega-3 fatty acids in fatty fish—have been connected to better mental health and a lower chance of developing depression. Consuming foods high in antioxidants, such as vibrant fruits and vegetables, can help shield brain tissue from oxidative stress, a condition linked to neurodegenerative illnesses and cognitive loss.

We will investigate the complex relationship between nutrition and mental health in more detail. We will go into the research underlying how different nutrients and dietary habits can affect your mood, mental health, and overall ability to think clearly. With this information, you will be able to make decisions about the foods you eat that will support your physical, emotional, and mental well-being.

A Quiet Supporter Against Illness

Food is a quiet partner in the fight against disease, in addition to being a means of nourishing our bodies and improving our mental and emotional health. Foods have the power to either build and boost our immune systems or weaken them, making us more vulnerable to a variety of illnesses.

Our immune systems can be weakened by an imbalanced diet deficient in vital nutrients, leaving us more susceptible to infections and long-term ailments. On the other hand, a diet high in antioxidants, vitamins, and minerals can give our immune systems the support they need to remain strong and prepared to fight off threats.

Furthermore, studies have demonstrated that particular meals have particular health-promoting qualities. For instance, garlic is well known for having antibacterial and anti-inflammatory qualities. Turmeric's strong anti-inflammatory and antioxidant properties are attributed to its main ingredient, curcumin. Eating these and similar foods can lower the chance of sickness and improve general health in a way similar to preventative medicine.

We shall examine these foods' health-promoting qualities and the science underlying them in "Food or Poison." We will also reveal the amazing synergy that exists between different dietary components and nutrients, showing how the appropriate combinations can function in unison to preserve and improve your health.

The Quest for Longevity

We will investigate how nutrition affects our longevity in-depth, going beyond short-term health benefits. We'll go to "Blue Zones," areas where a remarkably high proportion of individuals continue to live healthy lives well into their 90s and 100s. What distinguishes these locations? The lifestyle and mentality of the people who live in these distinct places, as well as their diet, are crucial factors.

Vegetables, fruits, nuts, and legumes are among the many plant-based foods that are consumed in Blue Zones, while processed meals and animal products are consumed in small amounts. We'll delve into the research underlying these dietary selections and how they support longer healthier lives.

We will also examine in depth the ideas of intermittent fasting and calorie restriction, two dietary practices that have demonstrated potential for improving health and prolonging life. Gaining knowledge about the research underlying these practices will help you maximize the potential of your diet to age gracefully and lead a longer, more satisfying life.

Making Informed Choices

We'll dispel myths and provide insight into the most recent findings in the field of nutrition research as we go. Distinguishing between nutritional fallacies and factual information is crucial to make well-informed dietary decisions.

We'll look at many dietary styles, such as Mediterranean and Paleo, as well as vegan and vegetarian, giving you an understanding of the benefits and possible downsides of each. With this knowledge, you will be able to make dietary decisions that support your beliefs and overall health objectives. We'll also go into the realm of food marketing and labeling, assisting you in understanding the frequently perplexing information found on food packaging. You'll learn what you need to know to confidently navigate the grocery store and make decisions that support your overall health and well-being.

The Power to Transform

As we go through the pages of this book, never forget that every meal you eat presents a chance for personal growth. The decisions you make at the dinner table speak volumes about your dedication to life, vitality, and health. You can shape a future of robust health and vibrant living with every mouthful.

In "Food or Poison," we set out on a scientific expedition to investigate the complex connection between our food decisions and overall health. This book serves as a resource for comprehending the science of nutrition, the effects that food has on our bodies and brains, and the opportunities for personal growth that each meal offers.

One bite at a time, you will learn to embrace the power you hold to design a future of robust health and bright well-being by keeping an open heart and an inquisitive mind. As we proceed through the pages of this book, get ready to gain knowledge, inspiration, and the ability to make decisions that will take care of your body, mind, and spirit.

The Trip Forward

We have only just begun our exploration, and there are many chances for growth and self-discovery along the way. Be ready to confront your beliefs as we delve further into the complex realm of nutrition, accept the facts backed by research, and discover the secrets to a healthier, happier life. Together, we will disentangle the nuances of nutrition and diet, from the fundamental components of food to the complicated relationships between nutrition, lifespan, and health. We'll examine how food affects our mental health, mood, and cognitive abilities while also illuminating the science underlying these connections.

We will explore the idea of food as a quiet ally against disease in the ensuing chapters, learning about the unique qualities of different foods and how they might strengthen our immune systems and prevent sickness. We'll also travel to the Blue Zones, where we'll investigate the nutritional practices that have helped the inhabitants live long, healthy lives. You'll discover the benefits of intermittent fasting and calorie restriction, two practices linked to longer lifespans, and how to incorporate them into your daily routine. We will guide you through the world of dietary patterns, covering everything from plant-based to Mediterranean, and provide you with the information you need to make wise dietary decisions.

Therefore, retain an open mind and a passion for information as we continue our exploration. With each chapter, you will gain a deeper understanding of the complex relationship between nutrition and health, giving you the confidence to take control of your health and use food as a catalyst for transformation.

CHAPTER 2
The Basics of Nutrition

The definitive guide to healthy eating in real life is to make little adjustments at first to consume a healthy diet. Aim to include nutrient-dense foods in every meal and snack, and stay away from processed foods.

What constitutes "healthy eating" varies depending on who you ask. Everyone appears to have an opinion about what constitutes a healthy diet, including coworkers, family members, wellness influencers, and healthcare professionals.

Furthermore, online nutrition articles can be quite confusing due to their contradicting recommendations and guidelines, many of which are incorrect. If all you want to do is eat in a way that is healthy and convenient for you, this makes it difficult.

In actuality, eating healthily doesn't have to be difficult. You can take care of your body and still enjoy the meals you love. Food is supposed to be enjoyed, not feared, measured, tracked, or counted.

Why is eating well important?

It's vital to discuss the importance of healthy eating before delving into what it entails.

First and foremost, food provides you with the energy and nutrition your body requires to function. Your health may suffer if you don't consume enough calories or certain nutrients in your diet.

Similarly, overindulging in calories can lead to weight gain. Obesity increases the risk of heart, liver, and renal problems, as well as type 2 diabetes and obstructive sleep apnoea.

Your longevity, mental well-being, and disease susceptibility are all impacted by the caliber of your nutrition. Diets primarily consisting of whole, nutrient-dense foods are linked to increased longevity and disease protection, whereas diets high in ultra-processed foods are linked to increased mortality and a greater risk of conditions like cancer and heart disease.

High-processed food diets may also raise the chance of developing depressive symptoms, especially in those with lower levels of physical activity. Additionally, you're probably not getting enough of some nutrients if your diet consists mostly of ultra-processed foods and drinks like soda, fast food, and sugary cereals and less whole foods like veggies, nuts, and fish. This could have a detrimental effect on your general health. Does eating healthily require you to adhere to a certain diet? Not! Most people don't need to adhere to any particular diet to feel their best, even though some people must—or choose—to avoid specific foods or adopt diets for health-related reasons.

That's not to argue that you can't gain from some eating habits. For example, although some people feel best on low-carb diets, others do best on high-carb diets. But generally speaking, following a diet or set of nutritional guidelines has nothing to do with eating healthily. "Healthy eating" is just putting your health first by supplying your body with wholesome nutrients. Each person's experience with the details may vary based on their location, socioeconomic status, social and cultural background, and personal preferences.

It's critical to comprehend the foundational ideas of nutrition to genuinely appreciate the effects of the foods we choose. This chapter, which examines the components that makeup life itself, is a pillar of our expedition.

Macronutrients: Fueling the Machine

Macronutrients, or the carbohydrates, proteins, and fats that make up the basis of our diet, are the essential components of every meal. In the complex dance of physiological processes, every one of these macronutrients has a specific and essential role to play.

Carbohydrates: The body's main source of energy, they are frequently unfairly vilified. Our cells, tissues, and organs are powered by glucose, which is produced when they are broken down. Simple carbs, like sugars, give you an immediate energy boost, but complex carbs, which are present in meals like whole grains, fruits, and vegetables, release energy gradually.

The distinction is comparable to that of a brightly lit but short-lived piece of paper against a slow-burning log on a fire that keeps you warm all night. I find that eating meals that include complex carbohydrates, such as sweet potatoes and brown rice, helps me stay energized all day.

Proteins: In charge of building and mending tissues, proteins are the builders of our bodies. They are made up of amino acids and are involved in many processes, ranging from immunological response to enzyme activity.

The body gets the building blocks it needs for development, maintenance, and repair when it consumes a varied diet of proteins.

For instance, I observed an improvement in my general muscle tone and strength during my workouts when I started integrating a range of protein sources like lean meats, seafood, lentils, and nuts into my diet. It also helped people recover from strenuous activity more quickly.

Water

Our bodies are made up of 45-75% water, which is essential for wellness. Water is utilized by the body for a variety of functions, including temperature regulation. Water, which is largely found in blood and other bodily fluids, aids in the movement of nutrients throughout the body and into and out of cells. Although the amount of water we require each day can vary based on factors like age and activity level, it's generally a good idea to consume 8 to 10 cups.

Fats: Although formerly believed to be detrimental to diet, fats are really necessary for a wide range of biological processes. They are essential for hormone synthesis, fat-soluble vitamin absorption, and the preservation of critical organs. Nuts, avocados, olive oil, and other foods high in healthy fats promote general health.

In my experience, eating foods high in healthy fats, such as nuts and avocados, not only made my food taste better but also helped me have skin and hair that are healthier. How relatively small adjustments may have such a significant impact on our well-being is amazing.

Micronutrients: The Unsung Heroes

While macronutrients are the main players, vitamins and minerals are the hidden heroes that make it possible for our bodies to operate at their best: micronutrients. These little substances are incredibly important to our health and well-being.

Vitamins: A variety of physiological functions depend on these chemical substances. Vitamins C and D, for example, assist bone health and the immune system, respectively, and each has a specific function to perform. A diversified diet makes sure that the body gets all the vitamins it needs.

When I decided to increase the diversity of fruits and vegetables in my diet, I can still clearly recall that time. My mood and general mental clarity seemed to have improved along with my immune system's strength. It felt like providing my body with the resources it required to function at its peak.

Minerals: Minerals are the foundation of all biological activity, from iron for oxygen transport to calcium for strong bones. They support nerve signaling, aid in fluid balance, and function as co-factors in enzyme activities. Meeting mineral requirements requires a varied diet high in fruits, vegetables, and whole grains.

I became aware of the significance of minerals directly when I began monitoring my iron consumption. I felt alert and more energized as a result, and my workouts got more efficient. It's incredible how little iron can seem to have such a significant impact on our emotions and behavior.

Deciphering the functions of macro- and micronutrients is like learning the language of life itself. It gives us the ability to make knowledgeable decisions about what we place on our plates, guaranteeing that we give our bodies the vital components they require to survive.

CHAPTER 3

The Modern Diet Dilemma

There are many different viewpoints and ideas on the complicated topic of the current nutrition conundrum. When making dietary decisions, it's critical to take into account several aspects, such as individual health objectives, ethical issues, and environmental impact. Let's examine some salient arguments from each side of the dispute:

1. **Medical Matters to Consider:**

Veganism: Proponents of this diet claim that a balanced plant-based diet may supply all the necessary nutrients for optimum health. Diets based mostly on plants tend to be lower in cholesterol and saturated fats, which can minimize the risk of heart disease and several cancers. On the other hand, vegans must be extremely mindful of their dietary intake, especially when it comes to vitamin B12, iron, calcium, and omega-3 fatty acids.

Diet Based on Meat: Iron, zinc, vitamin B12, and high-quality protein are among the vital elements found in meat. Lean meats can assist in providing these nutritional requirements in the diet. On the other hand, an increased risk of heart disease and some types of cancer has been linked to an excessive diet of red and processed meats.

2. Environmental and Ethical Considerations:

Veganism: A lot of people who practice veganism avoid eating anything that comes from animals because they care about the environment and animal welfare. They consider a plant-based diet to be more humane and sustainable.

Diet Based on Meat: Proponents of eating meat contend that it can be included in a balanced diet if it comes from sources that are ethical and sustainable. They might be in favor of methods like regenerative agriculture, which has a low impact on the environment.

3. Achieving Balance:

Flexitarianism: This diet consists mostly of plant-based foods, with the odd animal product. It provides more flexibility and maybe a more sensible choice for certain people who wish to cut back on meat consumption without giving it up entirely.

4. Personalized Method:

It's critical to understand that no one diet works for everyone. Every individual has different dietary requirements, tastes, and moral concerns. Making educated judgments based on their unique situation can be aided by speaking with a qualified dietitian or nutritionist.

A person's goals, values, and state of health all influence the "best" diet. When adopted thoughtfully, diets devoid of meat or dairy products can coexist with a healthy lifestyle. It's critical to concentrate on balanced nutrition, taking into account each person's needs while also being conscious of the moral and environmental ramifications of food choices. For individualized advice, speaking with a licensed dietician or other healthcare provider is advised.

Also, It might be difficult to navigate the sea of dietary trends in the constantly changing field of nutrition. There are seemingly countless options available for achieving maximum health and well-being, ranging from paleo to vegan to keto to Mediterranean. Let us address the ubiquitous problem of processed foods and their effects on our health, as well as the nuances of these dietary trends, analyzing their possible advantages and disadvantages.

The Varied Spectrum of Diets

As we explore this chapter, it is crucial to recognize the wide range of dietary strategies that people follow to improve their health. All of these diets—the plant-based, low-carb, high-fat Keto diet, the heart-healthy Mediterranean diet, or the ancestrally inspired Paleo diet—bring with them a distinct philosophy and nutritional emphasis.

Paleo Diet: The Paleo diet, which takes its cues from our ancestors, places a focus on whole, unprocessed foods including fruits, vegetables, nuts, and seeds, as well as lean meats and fish. Supporters of this diet want to replicate the eating patterns of early humans by avoiding processed foods, dairy products, and grains.

I tried the Paleo diet for a while and discovered that it inspired me to try a greater range of natural foods. It helped me become less dependent on junk snacks and rediscover my love for fresh fruit and lean meats.

Vegan Diet: The vegan diet, on the other hand, is a plant-based strategy that forgoes any animal products. An emphasis on fruits, vegetables, grains, legumes, nuts, and seeds is part of the movement to reduce their negative effects on the environment and to improve animal welfare.

My experience of trying a vegan diet was completely changed. It broadened my culinary horizons and made me more conscious of the ethical and environmental implications of food consumption. It forced me to think outside the box to satisfy my dietary requirements without using anything that comes from animals.

Keto Diet: The keto diet places a strong focus on eating a lot of fat, moderate amounts of protein, and few carbohydrates. The body enters a state of ketosis, when it largely uses fat for fuel, by dramatically lowering the amount of carbohydrates it consumes. Proponents assert advantages that include reduced body weight and enhanced mental clarity.

Although I didn't follow a strict keto diet, I did experiment with some of its components, including adding almonds and avocados, which are good fats, to my meals. I noticed that this change gave me longer-lasting energy and a fuller sensation, which helped me with my regular tasks.

Mediterranean Diet: This diet emphasizes entire foods, including fruits, vegetables, whole grains, fish, and olive oil. It is based on the cooking customs of the nations that border the Mediterranean Sea. It is well known for its ability to lengthen life and support heart health.

My general health started to improve as I started adopting a more Mediterranean-inspired strategy. My general vitality and energy levels seemed to improve when I included heart-healthy fats and a range of colorful fruits and veggies.

The Processed Food Pitfalls

The modern diet has become heavily reliant on processed foods due to our need for efficiency and convenience. These products, which are frequently loaded with harmful fats, processed sugars, and a myriad of artificial additives, can significantly affect our health.

When it comes to processed foods, discernment is essential. I've personally learned to carefully read labels and choose products with few ingredients and distinguishable constituents. This change not only made my nutrition better, but it also made a big difference in my energy and general sense of well-being.

Achieving Equilibrium

Remember that there is no one-size-fits-all approach to nutrition as we examine the wide variety of diets and struggle with the problems caused by processed meals. The most effective approach is frequently a customized blend of different dietary theories, adapted to specific tastes, health objectives, and ways of life.

I've learned through thoughtful decision-making and personal experimentation that the secret to long-term, sustainable well-being is to discover a balanced strategy that suits my body's requirements and preferences. It's about adopting an adaptable attitude and choosing deliberate actions that put fun and sustenance first.

It's important to approach dietary trends with an open mind in the always-changing field of nutrition, understanding that what works for one individual might not work for another. By being aware of the tenets and possible advantages of different diets, we enable ourselves to make decisions that will best support our path to optimum health and well-being.

CHAPTER 4

Food and diseases: What to know to ensure food safety

Notably, lately, we have begun to view foods. We have realized that food is very important as we eat it not only for the sake of energy and taste but also it helps us to stay fit and prevent diseases. But there are risks. People can also fall sick upon consuming food that has been prepared or handled incorrectly. We must learn about storing, cooking, and keeping food clean of germs for us to be certain that our food is safe at all times.

In some cases, food poisoning occurs when particular conditions are present. These factors include germ resistance; the number of germs present in a particular type of food, nutritional level of the individual consuming the food. Poor food may also have other aspects that might cause more damage to a person. Therefore, hygienic practices, such as thoroughly washing hands and ensuring proper clothing, are vital for employees when working on food.

This review provides a discussion on some of the main causes of ill health due to food. The most important microscopic organisms include bacteria, virus, parasite, fungus, and their poisonous byproducts. In addition, we discuss foods that trigger an allergy and intolerance. Some of these challenges are a result of how we preserve and store food for longer periods. A second way through which food can become unsafe.

Also, we discuss harmful additives that could be present in foods. Besides biology germs, it may include some chemicals such as pesticides and heavy metals. This can be harmful.

When talking about the safety of foods, it means their safety from the farm to our plates and this is what would help in keeping people safe from getting sick with whatever foods they eat. There are some safety measures that one should follow from the beginning to the end.

This chapter will examine the tremendous effects of diet on obesity, diabetes, and heart disease. It will also provide evidence-based insights into how particular dietary patterns can have a major impact on these disorders.

Heart Disease

Since heart disease is still one of the world's leading causes of death, there has been a lot of research done on how to prevent and treat it. It includes a wide spectrum of illnesses that impact the heart and blood arteries, such as arrhythmias, heart failure, and coronary artery disease. Public health must comprehend and treat the risk factors for heart disease.

Dietary Patterns and Cardiovascular Health: New research indicates that reducing the risk of cardiovascular disease is largely dependent on the diets we choose. Because of this, scientists and medical experts stress the need for dietary treatments to lower the incidence and severity of heart disease.

Saturated Fats and Cholesterol: Red meat, full-fat dairy products, and some processed meals are high in saturated fats, which are also associated with higher levels of LDL cholesterol, a key risk factor for heart disease. LDL cholesterol, sometimes known as "bad cholesterol," can build up in the arteries and cause atherosclerosis, a disorder that causes the blood vessels to shrink and stiffen. Heart attacks and strokes may become more likely as a result of this process. On the other hand, it has been demonstrated that replacing these sources with healthy fats—like the monounsaturated and polyunsaturated fats included in nuts, seeds, and fatty fish—improves lipid profiles. In the end, these "good fats" can help promote a healthier circulatory system by lowering LDL cholesterol and lowering the risk of atherosclerosis.

Dietary fiber: Whole grains, fruits, and vegetables are good sources of fiber, which is linked to lowered blood pressure and a lower risk of heart disease. There are several different types of fiber, both soluble and insoluble, and each has unique health advantages. For example, soluble fiber helps the body eliminate cholesterol by binding to its molecules in the digestive system. This activity helps to lower LDL cholesterol levels, which is important in lowering the risk of cardiovascular disease. Furthermore, fiber encourages fullness and aids in blood sugar regulation, both of which are critical components in preserving heart health. Eating foods high in fiber not only promotes cardiovascular health but also maintains a healthy gut flora, highlighting the complex relationship between gut and heart health.

Omega-3 Fatty Acids: Found in fatty fish such as salmon, mackerel, and walnuts, these important fatty acids have been shown to have anti-inflammatory qualities and have been repeatedly linked to a lower risk of heart disease. Atherosclerosis and other heart-related diseases are largely influenced by inflammation in their early stages of development and progression. The cardiovascular system can be protected by omega-3 fatty acids by reducing this inflammatory reaction. Moreover, they are essential for preserving normal blood vessel function and lowering the chance of arrhythmias, which are abnormal cardiac rhythms that can have dangerous repercussions. A heart-healthy diet plan should include the inclusion of foods high in omega-3s, or even supplements in certain situations.

public health must comprehend the complex relationship between nutrition and cardiac disease. Although dietary decisions are only one part of a complex strategy for managing and preventing heart disease, they are a potent way to lower risk and enhance cardiovascular health. Along with other lifestyle changes and medical therapies, the promotion of diets high in heart-healthy fats, fiber, and omega-3 fatty acids should continue to be a cornerstone of recommendations for cardiovascular health.

Diabetes

Millions of individuals worldwide suffer from diabetes, a metabolic disease that makes careful dietary management necessary to control blood sugar levels and avoid complications. An approach that is diverse and focuses on several dietary components is needed to achieve optimal control.

Carbohydrate Quality: When it comes to controlling blood sugar levels in people with diabetes, the kind and caliber of carbs ingested are crucial. Their diets should be centered on complex carbs from complete foods including vegetables, legumes, and whole grains. These foods encourage more stable glucose management since they have a slower effect on blood sugar levels. Additionally, they offer fiber, important minerals, and long-lasting energy, which makes them a smart option for those with diabetes.

Protein Intake: For those with diabetes, maintaining a balanced protein intake is essential. Protein maintains muscular function in addition to assisting in blood sugar stabilization. Fish, poultry, lentils, and tofu are examples of lean protein sources that are suggested to reduce the consumption of saturated fat. By selecting these protein sources, people with diabetes can lower their chance of cardiovascular problems and maintain a healthy body weight.

Glycemic Index: Knowing a food's glycemic index (GI) can help you better control your blood sugar levels. Foods are categorized by the GI according to how quickly they elevate blood sugar levels after ingestion. For people with diabetes, low-GI foods are recommended, such as sweet potatoes, quinoa, and most fruits. These low-GI foods help avoid sharp spikes and crashes in blood sugar levels by affecting them more gradually. By including them in the diet, you can encourage more consistent glucose regulation and lessen your need for prescription drugs or excessive insulin.

Apart from these dietary factors, effective management of diabetes also requires quantity control, meal scheduling, and customized meal planning. Speaking with a certified dietitian or other healthcare professional can offer individualized advice to address unique dietary requirements and guarantee that people with diabetes can have balanced, nutritious lives while lowering their risk of complications from their disease.

It's critical to keep in mind that there is no one-size-fits-all strategy for managing diabetes, and what works for one individual may not work for another. Therefore, customized eating regimens, frequent blood sugar checks, and a holistic approach to health are essential elements of effectively controlling diabetes.

Obesity

Because obesity is a serious health problem that has spread like an epidemic throughout the world, a great deal of research has been done to determine how nutrition affects both weight control and general health. Let's examine the complex network of variables that links diet to obesity in more detail.

Equilibrium Caloric:

The foundation of effective weight management is a balance between caloric intake and expenditure. This fundamental idea emphasizes how crucial it is to comprehend the energy equation, which pits calories in against calories out. A calorie deficit causes weight reduction, but consuming more calories than the body needs causes weight gain. Finding and keeping a healthy weight requires a careful balancing act between these two variables.

To attain this equilibrium, a diet high in nutrient-dense, whole foods is crucial. These meals offer a wealth of essential elements, such as vitamins, minerals, and antioxidants, in addition to calories, all without being overly high in empty calories. People can maintain their general health while controlling their calorie intake by selecting whole grains, lean proteins, and an abundance of fruits and vegetables.

Satiety and Portion Control: The ability to feel satisfied and full after eating is a key component of weight control. Foods that increase fullness can help manage portion sizes, avoid overindulging, and eventually support weight maintenance. Certain foods are known to have a satiating effect, especially those that are heavy in protein and fiber. Whole grains, legumes, and vegetables are examples of foods high in fiber that take longer to digest and keep you feeling fuller for longer. Likewise, hormones that indicate fullness and contentment are triggered by proteins. By incorporating these foods into your diet, you can improve the way you control your portion sizes.

Fried foods and sugar:

The current diet is full of highly processed foods and added sugars, both of which have been conclusively related to obesity and weight gain. Sugar-filled drinks, snacks, and desserts are high in calories and low in the vital nutrients that support fullness and general health. Consuming too much sugar can raise the risk of metabolic diseases, induce inflammation, and cause insulin resistance. It is important to minimize the consumption of these things to maintain a healthy weight and lower the risk of associated comorbidities.

Furthermore, trans fats, too much salt, and other additives found in highly processed foods might interfere with the body's normal appetite and satiety signals, causing overeating. Limiting the intake of processed foods and choosing complete, unprocessed substitutes can significantly influence weight control.

In conclusion, there is no denying the complicated yet clear link between nutrition and health, especially when it comes to heart disease, diabetes, and obesity. Numerous studies with strong evidence have shown definite links between food habits and the onset, course, and treatment of several illnesses. People can have a big impact on their health by choosing foods wisely and following balanced, nutrient-dense diets.

It's crucial to understand, though, that there isn't a one diet or method that works for everyone. It is essential to provide individualized food suggestions that take into account each person's tastes, health situation, and cultural background. Seeking advice from medical specialists, such as registered dietitians, can offer customized recommendations for enhancing eating patterns and advancing general health.

We shall examine the intricacies of dietary recommendations and realistic methods for incorporating a healthy diet into daily life in the upcoming chapter. These tactics will assist people in navigating the complicated world of nutrition and applying what they know about how eating affects health, which will eventually increase well-being and lower the risk of chronic illnesses like obesity.

CHAPTER 5

Food as Medicine

The significant role that food can play in promoting health and preventing disease has come to light more and more in recent years. The idea of "food as medicine" has received a lot of attention for its ability to improve human health, even though conventional treatment is still vital. This chapter will examine particular foods and how they can improve health as well as the newly popular idea of "functional foods" and their possible advantages.

The Healing Power of Food: Nourishing the Body, Mind, and Soul

Humans have needed food to survive from the beginning of time. But as we are starting to realize, eating is about more than just giving us energy and nourishment—some foods include ingredients and qualities that can improve our health and wellbeing. Now let's explore a few of these foods and their amazing health-boosting qualities:

1. Turmeric: This vibrant yellow spice, which is frequently used in curries, has a strong anti-inflammatory and antioxidant component called curcumin. Among its many advantages, curcumin has been connected to decreased inflammation and enhanced brain function. It might also have an impact on the avoidance of chronic illnesses.

2. Berries: Berries such as strawberries, blueberries, and others are rich in antioxidants, vitamins, and minerals. They may slow down aging since they have been linked to decreased oxidative stress and enhanced cognitive performance.

3. Fatty Fish: Omega-3 fatty acids, which are abundant in fish like salmon, mackerel, and sardines, have been demonstrated to lessen the risk of heart disease, reduce inflammation, and enhance brain function. It is believed that these lipids are necessary for general health.

4. Garlic: Garlic is well-known for its unique taste, but it also has powerful therapeutic benefits. It has been connected to lowered blood pressure, raised immune system performance, and better cholesterol levels. Allicin, the key ingredient in garlic, is the source of many of these health advantages.

5. Leafy Greens: Superfoods in terms of nutrition include collard greens, kale, and spinach. They include a lot of antioxidants, vitamins, and minerals. Eating them has been linked to a decreased chance of developing chronic illnesses, such as heart disease and several forms of cancer.

6. Probiotics: Good bacteria found in foods like yogurt, kefir, and fermented veggies help maintain gut health. Immunity, mental health, and digestion all depend on a healthy gut microbiota. Probiotics can assist in preserving this delicate equilibrium.

7. Nuts and Seeds: Walnuts, almonds, chia seeds, and flaxseeds are a great way to get fiber, important nutrients, and healthy fats. They have been connected to better weight control and a decrease in heart disease risk factors.

8. Bone Broth: Rich in collagen, gelatin, and amino acids, among other vital nutrients, bone broth promotes joint, skin, and intestinal health.

9. Berries (strawberries, raspberries, and blackberries): Rich in antioxidants, fiber, and vitamins, berries are great for brain and cardiovascular health.

10. Avocado: Rich in fiber, heart-healthy fats, and a variety of vitamins and minerals, avocados give you long-lasting energy.

11. Sweet potatoes: Rich in antioxidants, vitamins, and fiber, sweet potatoes help to balance blood sugar levels and support digestive health.

12. Probiotic-Rich Foods (Kefir, Kimchi, and Yogurt): These foods improve immunity and digestion by supporting a balanced gut microbiota.

13. Nuts and Seeds (Almonds, Chia Seeds, Flaxseeds): Rich in fiber, heart-healthy fats, and vital nutrients, these foods lower inflammation and support heart health.

15. Green tea: Packed with antioxidants, especially catechins, green tea promotes metabolic health and may provide some cancer-prevention benefits.

17. Mushrooms (Reishi, Shiitake, and Maitake): These fungi have been linked to better immune function and are rich in substances that strengthen the immune system.

18. Quinoa: Packed with fiber, vitamins, minerals, and vital amino acids, quinoa is a complete protein source.

19. Oats: Packed with fiber, oats promote healthy digestion and help control blood sugar levels.

20. Broccoli: Renowned for its general nutritional density and ability to combat cancer, broccoli is a vegetable rich in vitamins, minerals, and antioxidants.

21. Cabbage: Rich in vitamins, minerals, and phytochemicals that boost digestive health and immune system performance, cabbage is a cruciferous vegetable.

22. Lentils: Packed with fiber, folate, and other minerals, lentils are a fantastic plant-based protein source.

23. Chia seeds: Packed with fiber, omega-3 fatty acids, and other vital minerals, these small seeds are a powerhouse.

24. Pomegranate: Rich in antioxidants, pomegranates have been linked to decreased inflammation and better heart health.

25. Beets: Packed with nitrates and antioxidants, beets promote cardiovascular health and may improve athletic performance.

26. Cinnamon: A versatile spice with many health advantages, cinnamon is well-known for

its anti-inflammatory and anti-diabetic qualities.

27. Grapes: Packed with heart-healthy antioxidants like resveratrol, grapes may also have anti-aging qualities.

28. Sauerkraut: Similar to sauerkraut, fermented cabbage is a high-probiotic food that strengthens the immune system and promotes intestinal health.

29. Walnuts: Rich in antioxidants, omega-3 fatty acids, and other elements, these nuts are an excellent source of nutrition.

30. Seaweed (Nori, Kelp): Packed with iodine, vitamins, and minerals, seaweed promotes thyroid function and the health of the entire metabolic system.

31. Lemon: Rich in antioxidants and vitamin C, lemons help with digestion and immune system support.

Though these foods have many health advantages, keep in mind that you need to eat a varied and balanced diet to guarantee you get all the critical elements. Including a wide variety of therapeutic foods in your diet can be a significant step toward encouraging the best possible health and well-being. Before making major dietary changes, always get advice from a medical expert or trained dietician, particularly if you have any particular health issues.

These are but a handful of the numerous meals that can be effective partners in the pursuit of improved health. Their natural ingredients are crucial parts of a "food as medicine" strategy since they can prevent and treat a wide range of illnesses.

Foods with Functions: Not Just Nutrition

Even while every complete food has healthy nutrients, some foods are even more special since they are labeled as "functional foods." These are foods that, frequently because of certain bioactive substances they contain, offer health advantages above and beyond basic nourishment. Functional foods are made to actively aid in the treatment and prevention of several health problems in addition to simply sating hunger. The following are some instances of functional foods and possible health advantages:

1. Probiotic Yogurt: Live probiotic cultures added to yogurt enhance immune system health and digestion by preserving healthy gut flora. Additionally, it might lessen irritable bowel syndrome symptoms (IBS).

2. Oatmeal: Beta-glucans, a kind of soluble fiber with a reputation for lowering cholesterol, is found in oats. Regular oat consumption can help lower the risk of heart disease.

Green Tea: Catechins, potent antioxidants found in green tea, may help prevent cell damage and inflammation. It has been linked to enhanced cognitive performance and a lower incidence of specific types of cancer.

Soy-Based Products: Isoflavones, which are found in soy products like tofu and soy milk, may help lessen the symptoms of menopause and possibly even cut the risk of osteoporosis. Consuming soy has also been associated with a decreased risk of heart disease.

5. Cucumbers: Lycopene, an antioxidant found in tomatoes, has been shown in studies to lower the incidence of prostate cancer and promote heart health.

6. Supplements with Turmeric: As was previously established, curcumin, a compound found in turmeric, has strong anti-inflammatory effects. Supplements containing turmeric are frequently used to lessen inflammation and ease the symptoms of illnesses like osteoarthritis.

7. Foods fortified: Certain minerals, like folic acid in cereals and vitamin D in milk, are added to a lot of foods to make them more nutritious. These are intended to improve health and solve particular nutritional deficits.

Functional foods can play a crucial role in a comprehensive strategy for overall health and wellness since they are specifically formulated to provide these health advantages. It's crucial to remember that although functional foods can be a beneficial complement to a diet, a balanced, diverse, and nutrient-rich diet should always come first.

Using Food as Medicine in Everyday Living

Using the idea of food as medicine in our day-to-day activities is a proactive and empowering way to take care of our health and well-being. We can prevent sickness, support our bodies natural processes, and even manage specific health concerns by choosing foods that are good for us. The following are some doable methods to incorporate food's healing properties into our daily routines:

1.   **Accept Complete, High-Nutrient Foods**

The cornerstone of using food as medicine is giving full, nutrient-dense foods top priority. These are whole foods that are high in vital nutrients like vitamins, minerals, fiber, and antioxidants in their unprocessed, natural state. Your diet should be centered around fruits, vegetables, whole grains, lean proteins, and healthy fats. For a wide range of nutrients, try to eat a colorful assortment of fruits and veggies.

2. Conscientious Meal Scheduling

Plan meals that are well-balanced and contain a range of nutrients. Include a combination of micronutrients (minerals and vitamins) and macronutrients (proteins, fats, and carbohydrates). Aim to incorporate a varied variety of foods in your meals, taking into account the individual health advantages of each. For instance, choose omega-3-rich fatty seafood like salmon and include leafy greens because of their high vitamin and mineral content.

3. Unleash the Potency of Spices and Herbs

In addition to being flavor enhancers found in nature, herbs and spices have potent therapeutic properties. For instance, curcumin, which has anti-inflammatory qualities, is present in turmeric. Ginger is particularly good for digestion, while cinnamon can help control blood sugar levels. Try experimenting with different herbs and spices to improve the flavor of your food as well as its ability to promote health.

4. Make Gut Health a Priority

General health needs to have a healthy stomach. Consume foods high in probiotics, such as kefir, kimchi, sauerkraut, and yogurt, to help maintain a varied and harmonious gut flora. Prebiotic meals that feed good gut flora include onions, garlic, and vegetables high in fiber. Stronger immunity, better digestion, and even better mental health can all be attributed to a healthy gut.

5. Adjust to Your Specific Requirements

Take into account your health objectives as well as any dietary needs or limits you may have. For instance, if controlling blood pressure is your goal, concentrate on eating foods high in potassium, such as sweet potatoes, spinach, and bananas. Include calcium-rich foods like dairy products, fortified plant-based milk, and leafy greens in your diet to support bone health.

6. Keep Your Water Up

Our bodies are primarily made of water, which is necessary for circulation, digestion, and proper cellular operation. Sufficient water facilitates the body's capacity to assimilate and employ nutrients obtained from meals. In addition to making sure you get enough water throughout the day, think about consuming hydrating foods like celery, cucumbers, and watermelon.

7. Pay Attention to Your Body

Take note of your feelings after eating various foods. Take note of which foods give you energy and which make you feel bloated or lethargic. This self-awareness can help you choose foods that suit the particular requirements and preferences of your body.

8. Ask for Expert Advice

See a qualified dietician or other healthcare professional if you have any particular dietary needs or health concerns. They can offer you individualized guidance based on your unique situation and support you in overcoming any nutritional obstacles you may face.

Using food as medicine in daily life is a holistic approach to health that encourages people to actively participate in their health. We may maximize our nutrition, support our bodies natural processes, and ultimately improve our general quality of life by choosing foods with intention and thoughtfulness. Recall that each meal presents a chance to both nourish and repair the body, so make thoughtful choices and relish the advantages of this potent kind of self-care.

CHAPTER 6

Exposing Diet Myths: Dispelling 20 Common Misconceptions.

There is a lot of information available in the field of nutrition, and it can occasionally be difficult to separate reality from fiction. This chapter seeks to dispel some of the most widespread fallacies about diets, supported by research to assist you in making well-informed dietary decisions.

20 Common Myths About Diet

Myth 1: Carbs are the Enemy

The subject of carbohydrates and dieting has always been mistreated. However, in most cases, they are an important source of energy for the body. Natural carbohydrates such as nuts, fruits, salad vegetables, and whole grains are rich in vital vitamins, and fibers and slow energy supply. Refined and processed carbs should only be consumed in small quantities.

Myth 2: Eating Fat Makes You Fat

Dietary fat is a vital macro-nutrient, which has numerous roles in the body's function. Such avocados, nuts, seeds, and oils in the form of healthy fats promote a healthy heart, brain development, and general bodily functioning. Instead, it is essential to consider what types of fats are consumed.

Myth 3: Lose weight by skipping meals.

Missing meals may turn out to be counterproductive for losing weight. Well-balanced meals are essential for regularizing metabolic functions, maintaining stable blood sugar levels, and avoiding overeating at night. One must think about the diet every single time during the day.

Myth 4: All Calories Are Created Equal

Although calorie intake plays a role in weight control, the kind of calories ingested also matters. Healthy dietary practices include consuming nutritionally dense, whole foods that offer more than simple energy; additional vital vitamins, minerals, and antioxidants are required for optimal health.

Myth 5: You Must Detox or Cleanse Often.

The body has its natural detox mechanisms like the liver and kidneys, which are always busy removing wastes and toxins from the body. However, extreme detox diets or cleanses could be harmful, stripping the body of essential nutrition while producing unstable chemical imbalances.

Myth 6: You Can Spot-Reduce Fat

Contrary to common conception, isolated fat-burning exercises such as crunches or leg lifts do not target specific areas for fat loss. Fat is lost systematically in the body with the influence of factors such as genes, and total calories burnt.

Myth 7: Why eating late makes you fat.

The important thing is not when you eat but the number of calories consumed daily. However, late-time snacks cannot always be a problem as long as there is no excess eating. It is possible to have a healthy balanced meal or snack at night as well.

Myth 8: Gluten-Free Equals Healthier

Gluten avoidance is important for persons suffering from celiac disease or having gluten sensitivity. On the other hand, whole grains containing gluten such as wheat, barley, and rye can be beneficial for a larger audience. It is essential to eat whole untreated food instead of replacing it with other innutritious alternatives for gluten-free products.

Myth 9: All Protein Supplements are Equal

The quality of protein supplements greatly differs depending on their compositions. Although some may be good for people who need a certain diet or do intense exercises, the quality of these products should be great and you cannot consider them as the only product you take in food.

Myth 10: Eating Healthy is Expensive

Whole, unprocessed foods are an inexpensive way to maintain a balanced diet even when it comes to certain specialty health foods. Good quality items like beans, lentils, whole grains, and fruits in season are cost-effective items for a healthy meal.

Myth 11: Sugar Content Makes Fruit Bad.

These essential nutrients from fruit play a crucial role in ensuring optimal health. Fruit contains some very nutritious sugars. These are the added sugars that should not be consumed in excess.

Myth 12: Egg Yolks Should Be Avoided Due to Cholesterol.

The last several decades' studies suggest that blood cholesterol is not dependent upon dietary cholesterol. Nutrition-wise eggs hold vital proteins, vitamins, and mineral content. The inclusion of whole eggs into a diet may form part of a balanced healthy diet pattern.

Myth 13: Small and frequent meals increase metabolism.

Nevertheless, a change in the daily energy balance is modest concerning meal frequency. The balance of calories eaten per day and different foods are the essential elements.

Myth 14: Low-fat or fat-free products are always healthy.

Often, they replace lost fats in low-fat or fat-free products with added sugars or artificial flavors. However, some of these products are not necessarily the most appropriate health choice. Therefore, one should always look for labels and consider whole and unprocessed ones wherever suitable.

Myth 15: "All Plant-Based diets are healthful."

It should, however, be noted that while a well-balanced diet has the potential to be very nutritious, one can still choose low-quality foods even on a vegetarian diet. Plant-based food processing at high levels, overeating on candy, and lack of proper nutrition planning are common causes of such deficiency. A balanced approach is key.

Myth 16: Muscle building calls for high-protein diets"

Protein is necessary for the maintenance of muscle tissue but more does not mean more. A healthy diet, comprising of moderate proteins, is enough for most individuals including those involved in routine workouts as the body normally absorbs only a specified quantity of protein in the body.

Myth 17: Why natural sweeteners are better than regular sugar.

Refine sugar may contain a few additional nutrients found in natural sweeteners such as honey, maple syrup, or agave nectar, but it is also an added sugar that should be eaten sparingly by someone trying to manage their diet. The total amount of sugar should also be considered wherever it comes from.

Myth 18: You Need to 'Detox' from Sugar or Caffeine

Though limiting dependency may help in several cases, there is absolutely no need to go to extremes and follow full-blown detox protocols. Controlled and conscious consumption is a better way of managing intake compared to gradual reduction.

Myth 19: Low-Fat Dieting is Always the Healthiest Approach

It's vital to note that though saturated and trans fats are detrimental to the cardiovascular system, good fats should be incorporated into one's diet. Fats such as avocados, nuts, seeds, and olive oil are important to the functions of cells, regulators of hormones, and health.

Myth 20: You can out-exercise a poor diet.

Exercise helps in maintaining good overall health but you cannot outrun the bad diet. Nutrition and physical activity go hand in hand for gaining good weight and all-round health.

To sum up, dispelling popular diet myths is an essential first step toward choosing a sustainable and educated diet. We may empower ourselves to take a balanced, evidence-based approach to nutrition by learning to distinguish between reality and fiction, which will eventually improve our health and well-being. Remember that the cornerstone of lifelong health is a diet rich in whole foods. For individualized nutritional guidance catered to your unique requirements and circumstances, always seek the advice of a medical practitioner or registered dietitian.

CHAPTER 7

Mindful Eating and Portion Control

In a world where our fast-paced lifestyles regularly require us to multitask while eating, eat on the move, and frequently pay more attention to our devices than to our food, the idea of mindful eating appears as a glimmer of hope for a better connection with food. This chapter explores the significance of mindful eating and provides a wealth of useful advice on how to reduce portion sizes and prepare well-balanced meals that satisfy the senses and nourish the body.

The Deep Dive into the Art of Mindful Eating

Imagine this: you're eating dinner, but instead of shoving forkfuls of food into your mouth as you aimlessly browse around social media or watch TV, you approach your plate with reverence. Savoring every bite, you lose yourself in the harmonious blend of tastes, textures, and scents that tantalize your senses. You pay close attention to your body's cues about hunger and fullness and become intensely aware of these feelings.

This is what mindful eating is all about. It matters how much you eat as much as what you consume. During meals, this technique helps you to be fully present, establish a connection with the food on your plate, and pay attention to your body's cues. This is why it's so important:

1. **Enhanced Perceptual Experience**: Eating with awareness may turn an ordinary meal into a multisensory experience. It makes eating much more enjoyable by enabling you to recognize the subtle intricacies of every dish. You too can enjoy the rich experience of your meals, much as a gourmet chef or connoisseur might enjoy a beautiful wine or dish.

As an illustration, consider biting into a ripe, juicy strawberry. You take the time to properly taste it rather than just blindly chewing and swallowing it. You taste the delicious juiciness, the faint acidity, and the rush of sweetness. You will appreciate the strawberry more if you pay attention to it, and you might even discover that one or two will fulfill your demands.

2. **Improved Digestion:** Eating mindfully encourages you to chew your meal well, which improves digestion. This guarantees that your body can properly process the food and absorb the nutrients it contains, so it's more than

simply good manners. Additionally, healthy digestion lowers the chance of discomfort and bloating.

Picture a filling salad with bright veggies, crunchy greens, and an assortment of toppings. You are aiding your digestive system by breaking down complex fibers and plant chemicals with each bite that you chew thoroughly. This implies that after the meal, your stomach won't have to work as hard and you're less likely to feel bloated or heavy.

3. **Weight Control**: Mindful eating is a lifesaver if you have ever battled with weight management. Gaining more awareness of your body's hunger and fullness cues will help you prevent overindulging. Additionally, eating mindfully promotes a better connection with food that is unrestricted by emotional or impulsive eating.

At a dining table, for example, imagine yourself enjoying a delicious meal of spaghetti. You take a nibble or two to gauge how full you are, rather than just eating everything on the plate. You finish three-quarters of the meal and find yourself satiated. You've saved yourself from needless calories and that awkward "food coma" feeling by paying attention to your body.

4. **Emotional Consumption**: When we're anxious or depressed, many of us feel the impulse to grab comfort food. Encouraging you to face these emotional eating triggers is mindful eating. It asks you to identify instances in which you eat to sate your bodily hunger or to calm your emotional state.

Consider a day when you had extreme stress. When you're about to grab a bag of chips, you stop and consider whether you're hungry. If not, you're more inclined to look for better stress-reduction techniques, like going for a quick walk or practicing meditation.

5. **Moderate Satisfaction**: You're more likely to choose meals that satiate your urges when you eat mindfully. Smaller quantities may result from this, which may make it simpler to stop overindulging in harmful foods or excessive snacking.

Consider grabbing a piece of decadent, smooth chocolate cake. You take your time eating it, savoring every bite. The rich flavor and texture transform into an opulent encounter. You discover that a smaller slice fulfills your want for sweetness and leaves you feeling content without the need for a second dish.

Achievable Techniques for Mindful Consumption and Portion Management:

1. Delight in the Symphony: Reduce the speed at which you eat so that you can fully enjoy the tastes, textures, and fragrances of your food. Between mouthfuls, set down your utensils, chew well, and give your full attention to the food.

2. Respect Both Fullness and Hunger: Consider how hungry you are for a second before you eat. Are you motivated by boredom, tension, or habit, or are you genuinely hungry? Take regular breaks during the meal to assess your level of fullness. This maintains your awareness of your body's cues.

3. Reduce Distractions: Set aside a special area free from electronic devices for your meals. Put your phone away, turn off the TV, and sit down at a table with only your food in front of you.

4. Make Your Servings the Correct Size: Choose smaller bowls and plates so that you might feel fuller with less food because they give the appearance of greater quantities.

5. Plan Your Meals: Make thoughtful decisions by preparing meals and snacks ahead of time. Making a plan supports your nutritional objectives and keeps you away from rash, unhealthy decisions.

6. Conscious Food Buying: When you go grocery shopping, try to be mindful. Make a list and follow it, despite the temptation to indulge in junk food or foods that don't fit your dietary goals.

7. Be Totally into the Cooking Process: Use all of your senses when preparing food. As you prepare, take in the aromas of the ingredients and the food, and enjoy the process of making your meals.

8. Ritual of Gratitude: Give thanks for a moment before you eat. Consider the path that your food takes from the farm to the table. This easy habit cultivates gratitude and a healthy relationship with food.

9. Distinguish True Hunger from Emotional Cravings: Develop an understanding of the distinction between emotional and bodily cravings. If you're not hungry yet find yourself needing food, consider finding other ways to deal with stress or underlying emotions.

10. Hydration Check: Your body may occasionally indicate thirst rather than hunger. Drink a glass of water before reaching for a portion of food to make sure you're not just thirsty.

11. Ask for Expert Advice: If portion management and mindful eating are difficult for you, think about speaking with a mental health or qualified dietitian. They can offer tailored tactics and assistance to make your journey easier.

Creating Well-Balanced Meals: A Culinary Journey:

A nutritious diet's cornerstone is a balanced diet, which makes sure you get all the important nutrients in the right amounts at the right times. Here's a closer look at the guidelines for preparing well-balanced meals:

1. Sound of the Food Group: Fruits, vegetables, nutritious grains, lean Food Group Symphony meats, and healthy fats are the components of a balanced diet. Every category provides special nutrients that are essential for general health and energy.

As an illustration, visualize a dinner plate as a palette for a painter. It has a colorful assortment of veggies, a portion of lean protein, such as grilled chicken, quinoa (a whole grain), and a drizzle of healthy fat, and olive oil. This well-balanced combination provides a symphony of nutrients, including heart-healthy monounsaturated fats from olive oil, complex carbs in the quinoa, vital amino acids in the protein, and vitamins and minerals in the vegetables.

2. Mastery of Visual Portioning: Using visual signals in addition to accurate food measurement is essential for achieving portion control. A serving of whole grains should be about the size of your clenched fist, whereas a serving of lean protein should be about the size of your palm.

Consider a bowl of porridge with fresh berries on top as a normal breakfast. A serving of carbs that is roughly the size of your closed fist is what you should strive for when you scoop the oats into the dish. The berries on top enhance your meal by adding nutrients and flavor.

3. Whole Foods Are Everything: The main ingredients in your meals should be healthy foods like lean proteins, unprocessed whole grains, and fresh fruits and vegetables. They supply vital vitamins, minerals, and

antioxidants and are high in nutrients and low in calories.

Consider a salad that embodies the vibrant hues of summer. You heap grilled salmon, cherry tomatoes, sliced bell peppers, and crisp, dark greens on your dish. These complete, unprocessed meals are a veritable gold mine of vitamins and minerals that help you maintain good health and control your calorie consumption.

4. Equilibrated Macronutrients: There should be a balance of carbohydrates, proteins, and fats in every meal. Proteins aid in the healing of muscles and tissues, carbohydrates provide energy, and healthy fats are involved in several body processes.

A turkey and avocado sandwich on whole-grain bread is a staple lunch option. The avocado offers healthy fats that encourage satiety and nourish your body, the bread supplies carbohydrates for energy, and the turkey is full of lean protein for muscle repair.

5. The Part Fiber Plays: High-fiber foods including fruits, vegetables, and whole grains should be a part of every meal. In addition to helping with digestion and offering an

abundance of vitamins, minerals, and antioxidants, fiber also promotes feelings of fullness.

Think about having a vibrant stir-fry for supper. A variety of veggies, whole grain brown rice, and plant-based protein source tofu sizzling in your wok. Brown rice and vegetables' fiber helps you feel fuller so you can enjoy your food without going overboard.

6. Limit Sugar-Added Foods and Processed Foods: Processed foods can interfere with portion management and healthy eating since they contain hidden ingredients and empty calories. Reduce their presence in your diet to keep your calorie intake under control.

Consider your midday munchies. You grab a bowl of Greek yogurt with fresh honey and a sprinkle of nuts instead of a pre-packaged, sweet granola bar. This option offers a whole-food, balanced snack with less added sugar and empty calories.

7. The Key is Moderation: This balance rule applies to all foods. Although they have a role in your diet, even those less healthful options shouldn't take center stage during meals. Eat

them sparingly, appreciating them as the rare pleasure that they are.

Let's say you decide to treat yourself to a slice of your favorite rich, creamy cheesecake on a special occasion. Instead of feeling bad, you enjoy every bite because you know that this indulgent delicacy is a pleasant addition to your culinary adventure even though it's not something you do every day.

8. Maintain Hydration: An essential component of your food plan is water. Sufficient hydration promotes proper digestion, nutrient delivery, and waste elimination from the body, all of which are critical for general health.

*Consider a bright day when you're having grilled fish, steaming veggies, and a refreshing glass of cold water for dinner. * The water is the perfect beverage to keep you nourished and rejuvenated because it hydrates your body and goes well with your food.*

You go on a unique gastronomic trip toward a better and more balanced life by incorporating mindful eating habits and perfecting the art of portion control. These methods foster a strong bond with your food and a great appreciation for the eating experience. In addition to nourishing your body, balanced meals enchant your taste buds, allowing you to fully enjoy each dish.

It's your journey to portion control and mindful eating. It's about developing a relationship with food that is aware, appreciating its subtle sensory qualities, and savoring the flavors that dance across your tongue. It all comes down to making meals that are a symphony of flavors and minerals and selecting foods that genuinely nourish and fulfill. You are appreciating the poetry of your meals, one mouthful at a time, by practicing mindful eating and portion control.

CHAPTER 8

Customized Nutrition: Creating a Diet That Is Unique to You

The one-size-fits-all theory of nutrition has given way to a more sophisticated understanding in recent years: individualized nutrition. This new area recognizes that dietary requirements vary across individuals and are impacted by lifestyle, genetics, and personal preferences. We'll explore personalized nutrition in this chapter and see how it can completely change the way we think about diets.

The Personalized Nutrition Foundations

1. Genetic Difference:

Our bodies' nutrition use and metabolization processes are greatly influenced by our genes. There are genetic variants that can affect the way we metabolize proteins, lipids, and carbs. For instance, some people may benefit more from a lower-carb diet than others because they are more sensitive to carbohydrates. Analysis and testing based on genetics can shed important light on these differences.

2. Healthy Metabolism:

There can be significant individual variations in parameters such as cholesterol levels, insulin sensitivity, and metabolism rate. Comprehending these distinct metabolic characteristics enables customized food suggestions that promote maximum well-being.

3. Allergies and Food Sensitivities:

Personalized nutrition considers individual food sensitivities or allergies that may impact a person's capacity to process or endure particular foods. It is essential to stay away from these triggers for general well-being.

4. Activity and Lifestyle Levels:

Whether a person is sedentary, moderately active, or extremely active, it directly affects how much energy and nutrition they require. For example, athletes may require more protein and calories to support their training schedule.

5. Health Digestive:

Digestion enzyme levels can vary throughout people, which can have an impact on how well they digest and absorb nutrients from various diets. To guarantee adequate nutrient absorption, personalized nutrition takes these elements into account.

Putting Personalized Nutrition into Practice

1. Optimizing Macronutrient Ratios:

Understanding unique genetic differences connected to nutrition is now feasible because of developments in genetic testing. Businesses make individualized suggestions based on genetic predispositions through DNA analysis.

2. Evaluations of Nutritiousness:

For a thorough assessment of a person's nutritional requirements, speaking with a licensed dietitian or nutritionist might be beneficial. This covers elements including basal metabolic rate, dietary deficits, and targeted health objectives.

3. Food Log and Monitoring:

Maintaining an in-depth food journal can help identify trends in eating patterns and facilitate customized changes. By tracking nutrient consumption and highlighting possible areas for improvement, this approach can assist in identifying issue areas.

4. Rendering and Input:

There is frequently some trial and error involved in personalized nutrition. People might have to experiment with various food strategies and observe how their bodies react. Getting regular input and making necessary revisions is essential to creating the best-customized plan.

Practical Applications of Personalized Nutrition

1. Optimizing Macronutrient Ratios:

Personalized nutrition can optimize the proportion of carbs, lipids, and proteins to support energy levels, weight management, and general well-being based on individual needs.

2. Controlling Sugar Levels in Blood:

Personalized nutrition can help people with diabetes or insulin resistance stabilize their blood sugar levels by controlling their carbohydrate intake and planning the timing of their meals and snacks.

3. Customizing Micronutrient Consumption:

Personalized suggestions can target specific nutrient needs, such as maintaining appropriate levels of vitamin D, calcium, or iron.

4. Taking Care of Digestive Problems:

For those suffering from disorders like lactose intolerance, celiac disease, or irritable bowel syndrome (IBS), personalized nutrition can help identify and steer clear of trigger foods.

5. Aiding with Weight Control:

Personalized strategies can be developed to assist people in reaching and maintaining a healthy weight following their metabolic profile, degree of exercise, and food preferences.

The Future of Nutrition: Empowering Individuals

Personalized nutrition signifies a revolutionary change in the way we approach our eating habits. Acknowledging the diversity of our nutritional needs helps us to go beyond general dietary recommendations and into a more personalized space where each person's genetic composition, lifestyle, and tastes are the focus. This gives people the power to choose diets that are both sustainable and suited to their health and well-being.

Collaboration between patients, medical providers, and nutrition scientists is necessary to implement individualized nutrition in our daily lives. We may anticipate more advanced instruments and technologies to further hone individualized food suggestions as the field develops.

In the end, nutrition will come from appreciating and celebrating our uniqueness; in the future, our food will genuinely represent who we are and help us to live long healthy lives.

The Practical and Ethical Aspects of Tailored Nutrition

1. Implications for Ethics:

Personalized nutrition presents ethical questions even though it has enormous promise to improve health. It is imperative to ensure fair access to genetic testing and individualized nutritional guidance for all individuals, irrespective of their socioeconomic situation.

2. Cultural Sensitivity:

Customized nutrition needs to be mindful of cultural differences in eating customs and preferences. Instead of imposing a uniform strategy, it needs to honor the diverse range of international culinary customs.

3. Vertical Sustainability

Personalized nutrition needs to be long-term sustainable to be genuinely beneficial. Rather than depending on band-aid solutions, it ought to enable people to make wise decisions and cultivate a positive relationship with food.

4. Healthcare Integration:

To provide accurate and useful individualized dietary advice, healthcare professionals—such as dietitians, doctors, and genetic counselors—must collaborate. This integrated approach guarantees a thorough comprehension of each person's healthcare requirements.

5. Eternal Investigations and Progress:

Personalized nutrition will continue to develop as our knowledge of metabolism, genetics, and nutritional science expands. To optimize the advantages of this strategy, it will be crucial to stay current with emerging research and technological advancements.

Putting Customized Nutrition into Practice: A Step Towards Holistic Health

In our pursuit of optimum health and well-being, personalized nutrition marks a substantial advancement. It recognizes the complex interactions that exist between our genetic composition, way of life, and personal preferences. By adopting this strategy, we take a step toward a day when nutrition serves as a potent instrument for flourishing in all facets of our lives rather than just providing for our basic needs.

Personalized nutrition can completely change the way we approach our diets as it becomes more widely available and sophisticated. It gives us the ability to control our health in a way that is uniquely suited to each of us. Remember that developing a sustainable, balanced eating plan that promotes your general well-being is the goal of personalized nutrition, not perfection.

We'll look at doable tactics in the upcoming chapters to help you incorporate tailored nutrition into your everyday routine. You'll set out on a quest to become a more vibrant and nourished version of yourself, from discovering your genetic predispositions to making educated food decisions.

CHAPTER 9

Selecting Sustainable Foods

Does what we eat have an impact on the environment? Yes, scientists agree. Diets heavy in animal protein and some crops can emit methane and other emissions from burning fossil fuels into the environment, use more water, and deplete the soil. Large-scale farming techniques that need a lot of resources are necessary for raising cattle and agriculture. A sustainable diet, on the other hand, can decrease these effects and the environmental damage caused by agriculture.

The concept of food sustainability can lessen the effects of climate change on the environment, human health, and welfare the more people embrace it.

Sustainable Eating: What Is It?

Eating sustainably refers to selecting food items that include the effects of production on soil, water use, pesticides, clearing land, greenhouse gas emissions, and the use of fossil fuels. When choosing what to eat, people who practice sustainable eating look for foods that come from farming methods that are as environmentally friendly as possible.

Eating sustainably affects more than just the environment. It is also generally acknowledged to be more nutrient-dense than a traditional diet.

Elements of a Diet That Are Sustainable

The main components of a sustainable diet are fruits, vegetables, legumes, whole grains, and some nuts. It stays away from most processed foods, including refined carbohydrates and sugar. Fish and meat raised and harvested with consideration for the environment can be considered sustainable foods. But since red meat—especially beef—contributes significantly to methane emissions and land destruction, it is not seen as sustainable.

Advantages of a Sustainable Food Plan

Because legumes and grains are less expensive to produce and need fewer resources than cattle, eating sustainably is less expensive than consuming a diet high in meat. Nutrient content is high in these foods. They can aid in the prevention of long-term conditions including high blood pressure, which has been connected to a diet heavy in processed foods and red meat.

Eco-Friendly Cooking Techniques

Understanding how contemporary agriculture affects the environment and climate change is the first step toward implementing sustainable food practices. People won't be able to choose the food they buy and eat with knowledge until then. Just like with everything new, it can be challenging to know where to start. Determining whether implementing sustainable eating practices as a component of the climate change solution can also be challenging.

Sustainable agriculture is a necessary topic to bring up while talking about sustainable food practices. By lowering the demand for beef, some sustainable lifestyle choices, such as eating little to no red meat, can lower methane emissions. Conventionally grown fruits, nuts, and vegetables also need a lot of chemicals and water.

So, in our pursuit of sustenance, we must acknowledge that the effects of the foods we choose to eat go beyond our health. Our food choices have a significant impact on the environment, impacting things like biodiversity, climate change, and resource use.

Food's Environmental Footprint

1. Emissions of Carbon

The transportation, processing, and production of food all have a major impact on greenhouse gas emissions. Methane emissions from livestock farming, particularly the production of beef, are a significant factor. Food goods transported over vast distances also contribute to the carbon footprint.

2. Deforestation and Land Use

Large-scale agriculture frequently results in habitat degradation and deforestation, especially when it comes to animal husbandry. This lowers the planet's ability to absorb carbon dioxide and disturbs ecosystems.

3. Use of Water

There is a huge water requirement in the production of several goods, like dairy and meat. Especially when it comes to livestock production, water usage is significant. Furthermore, aquatic habitats may suffer as a result of agricultural runoff polluting waterways.

4. Loss of Biodiversity

Large-scale monoculture farming methods can result in a loss of biodiversity since they concentrate resources on a single crop. This is because fewer habitats are available for various species to flourish.

How to Choose Sustainable Foods

1. Give Plant-Based Options Priority

Diets high in plant-based foods are much less harmful to the environment than diets high in animal products. Increased consumption of fruits, vegetables, legumes, and whole grains can help you drastically lessen your influence on the environment.

2. Select Seasonal and Local Foods

Whenever feasible, choose foods that are produced locally. Because they require less transportation, they produce fewer carbon emissions during long-distance shipment. Eating in season also lessens the need for energy-intensive greenhouse production and promotes local agriculture.

3. Reduce Food Wastage

Global food production wastes about one-third of its food supply. You may contribute to the reduction of this startling number by paying attention to portion sizes, keeping food properly, and finding new uses for leftovers.

4. Encourage Sustainable Agricultural Methods

Look for "organic," "fair trade," or certificates from bodies like the Marine Stewardship Council or the Rainforest Alliance. Products with these labels follow specific ethical and environmental guidelines.

5. Decrease Meat Intake

While going vegetarian or vegan is one strategy, cutting back on meat consumption can also be beneficial. When it comes to meat, think about eating more vegetarian meals and selecting lean meats that come from sustainable sources when you do.

6. Thoughtful Seafood Selections

An important danger to ocean ecosystems is overfishing. Select seafood that comes from sustainable sources and is, if possible, certified by agencies such as the Marine Stewardship Council.

7. Reduce the Amount of Processed Foods

Producing and packing processed goods frequently uses more energy and resources. Choosing whole, minimally processed foods is better for the environment and your health at the same time

8. Adopt Sustainable Practices and Local Farmers

Look for local food co-ops, farmers' markets, and community-supported agriculture (CSA) initiatives. These choices frequently emphasize ecologically friendly and sustainable methods.

9. Adopt a Conscientious Consumerist Lifestyle

Learn about the brands and businesses you endorse. Examine their adherence to environmental conservation, ethical standards, and sustainability practices.

10. Teach Others and Yourself

Keep up with food and environmental news. Knowing the consequences of the food you eat allows you to make more thoughtful selections and can encourage others to follow suit.

Final Thought: Nourishing the Earth, Nourishing Ourselves

Not only may our dietary choices affect our health, but they can also impact the health of the world. Adopting sustainable eating habits makes us stewards of a more harmonious and balanced coexistence of humans and the natural world. A more sustainable future is just one tiny but important step away from us with every thoughtful decision we make, such as choosing to eat locally and prepare plant-based meals. Let the food we eat be a catalyst for good in the world we live in and the place we call home.

CHAPTER 10

Implementing Positive Changes

Making the shift to healthier eating habits is a significant step toward increased vitality and well-being. The goal of this chapter is to give you useful advice and methods for incorporating these constructive adjustments into your day-to-day activities. Through a holistic approach and deliberate decision-making, you can develop enduring habits that promote your long-term well-being.

1. Gradual Progression over Quick Fixes

Rather than coming from abrupt, dramatic shifts, sustainable change frequently results from small, incremental changes. Focus on building a foundation of healthy, balanced decisions that you can sustain over time, rather than chasing quick fixes.

2. Set Realistic, Specific Goals

Establish attainable goals that are specific to your needs and tastes. Whether it's increasing the amount of vegetables in your meals or cutting back on sugary snacks, having clear goals gives you focus and inspiration.

3. Prioritize Whole, Unprocessed Foods

Place a focus on whole foods, such as whole grains, fruits, vegetables, lean meats, and healthy fats. These nutrient-dense foods serve as the foundation of a balanced diet by offering important minerals, vitamins, and antioxidants.

4. Mindful Meal Planning and Preparation.

Make time to organize and cook meals ahead of time. This not only guarantees that you have wholesome options close at hand but also lessens the probability of impulsive, unwise decisions.

5. Diversify Your Plate

To guarantee a wide range of nutrients, include a diverse range of foods. Try varying the fruits, veggies, whole grains, and proteins in your meals to make them nutrient-dense and engaging.

6. Practice Portion Control

Pay attention to portion proportions to avoid overindulging. To determine the right serving sizes for proteins, cereals, and vegetables, use visual clues such as the size of your palm or a deck of cards.

7. Keep Your Water Up

Maintaining adequate hydration is critical to general health and well-being. Make a conscious effort to stay hydrated throughout the day by drinking enough water. Sparkling water, flavored water, and herbal teas can all be tasty substitutes.

8. Pay Attention to Your Body

Observe your body's signals of hunger and fullness. Consume food only when you're hungry, and quit when you're full. This introspective method promotes a more intuitive connection with food.

9. Eat in a Balanced Way

Aim for well-balanced meals that include a variety of macronutrients, such as proteins, fats, and carbohydrates. A balanced plate encourages satisfaction and long-term energy.

10. Incorporate conscious eating.

When eating, use every sense in your body. Enjoy your food's scents, tastes, and textures. Chew mindfully, taking your time so you can enjoy every bite of the food and the occasion.

11. Make a Snack and Treat Schedule

Prepare for times when you might feel like having a snack or treat, and always have wholesome options on hand. This proactive strategy aids in averting snap decisions that are unhealthy.

12. Acclimate to Environmental and Social Factors

Take a flexible stance when it comes to eating. Make deliberate decisions that support your overall health goals, whether dining out or in social settings, while having fun.

13. Remain educated and mindful.

Continue your education regarding health and nutrition. Keep an open mind and be willing to try new foods, recipes, and dietary methods that suit your tastes and health objectives.

14. Establish a helpful environment.

Encircle yourself with people who share your goals when it comes to health. This network of support can provide motivation, responsibility, and insightful information about your path.

15. Exercise patience and self-compassion.

Recognize that changing for the better is a process rather than a destination. Be patient and kind to yourself, acknowledging your accomplishments and taking lessons from any difficulties you may have had.

16. Recognize Your Successes

No matter how tiny, recognize and celebrate your accomplishments. Acknowledging your accomplishments strengthens your resolve to keep up the beneficial lifestyle adjustments you have made.

Final Thoughts: A Path of Self-Care and Nourishing

Making healthy dietary adjustments is a significant self-care practice that demonstrates your dedication to overall well-being. By incorporating these doable tactics into your everyday routine, you open the door to long-term health and vitality. Recall that progress, not perfection, is what matters—a path of sustenance that helps you live the healthiest, most fulfilling life possible. Accept each step as a journey towards long-lasting health and happiness, guided by the transformative power of a mindful diet.

CHAPTER 11

Recipes and Meal Plans

This chapter provides some great sample meal plans that are tailored specifically for different dietary needs. The recipes prefer unrefined foods with varied tastes in flavor and texture. From vegetarian and protein diets to simple meals, there is something for everyone looking for recipe ideas from various destinations in Southeast Asia.

Recipe 1: Mediterranean Chickpea Salad

Ingredients:

- 1 can (15oz) of drained and rinsed chickpeas
- 1 cup cherry tomatoes, halved
- 1 cucumber, diced
- 1/2 red onion, finely chopped
- 1/4 cup fresh parsley, chopped
- 1/4 cup feta cheese (optional)
- 2 tablespoons olive oil
- 2 tablespoons lemon juice

- Salt and pepper to taste

Instructions:

1. Place chickpeas, cherry tomatoes, cucumber, red onion, and parsley into a large bowl.
2. It can be garnished with some Feta cheese if necessary.
3. Put olive oil, lemon juice, salt, and pepper in a small bowl and whisk it together.
4. Lightly drizzle with the dressing, and toss lightly to coat all of the salad.
5. Serve chilled.

RECIPE 2: LEMON-DILL SAUCE WITH GRILLED SALMON.

Ingredients:

- 2 salmon fillets
- 2 tablespoons olive oil
- Salt and pepper to taste
- For the sauce:
- 1/4 cup Greek yogurt
- 1 tablespoon fresh dill, chopped

- 1 tablespoon lemon juice
- 1 teaspoon honey
- Salt to taste

Instructions:

1. Set the grill at a medium-high temperature and allow it to warm up.
2. Salt and pepper Olive oiled Brush salmon fillets.
3. Salmon should be grilled for approximately 4-5 minutes per side or until it breaks into flake-like small pieces when you try to insert a fork in it.
4. Combine Greek yogurt with dill, lemon juice, honey, and just a pinch of salt in a small bowl for the sauce.
5. Serve the grilled salmon together with the dab of lemon-dill sauce.

Recipe 3: Mushroom and Spinach Stir - Fry (Vegetarian Diet)

Ingredients:

- 2 cups mushrooms, sliced
- 3 cups fresh spinach
- 1 bell pepper, thinly sliced
- 1 small onion, thinly sliced

- 2 cloves garlic, minced
- 2 tablespoons soy sauce
- 1 tablespoon sesame oil
- 1 teaspoon ginger, grated
- Serve with cooked brown rice or quinoa.

Instructions:

1. In a large skillet or wok, heat the sesame oil on a high-medium fire.
2. Saute the garlic and ginger for about half a minute till aromatic.
3. Put in some mushrooms, bell peppers, and onions. stir-fry for 5-7 minutes for tender vegetables.
4. Add spinach and soy sauce and continue cooking for another 2 – 3 minutes until the spinach is softening.
5. Then serve it with cooked brown rice or quinoa.

SAMPLE MEAL PLAN:

Day 1:

Breakfast: Strawberry, blueberries, and walnut Greek yogurt parfait.

Lunch: Mediterranean Chickpea Salad

Dinner: Salmon on the grille with lemon-dill sauce served with steamed broccoli and quinoa.

Day 2:

Breakfast: Spinach and Mushroom Omelette with whole-grain toast

Lunch: Brown rice stir-fried mushrooms and spinach.

Dinner: Mixed green salad with balsamic vinaigrette and vegan lentil soup.

Day 3:

Breakfast: Avocado Toast with poached eggs

Lunch: Caprese Salad with balsamic glaze

Dinner: Chickpea and Vegetable Curry with basmati rice

Day 4:

Breakfast: Overnight Chia Pudding with mixed berries and almonds

Lunch: Quinoa and Black Bean Stuffed Bell Peppers

Dinner: Roasted chicken breast with sweet potatoes and asparagus.

Day 5:

Breakfast: Whole Grain Pancakes with maple syrup and sliced bananas

Lunch: Spinach and Feta Salad with balsamic vinaigrette

Dinner: Vegan Lentil Curry with brown rice

Day 6:

Breakfast: Greek yogurt smoothie with spinach, pineapples, and protein powder

Lunch: Lemon-Tahini Dressing on Chickpea and Avocado Salad

Dinner: Quinoa and steamed green beans accompanied by grilled Portobello mushrooms

Day 7:

Breakfast: Sautéed Spinach, Scrambled Eggs and Cherry Tomatoes

Lunch: Whole wheat turkey and avocado wrap.

Dinner: Baked salmon with garlic butter sauce, roasted Brussels sprouts, and wild rice.

Day 8:

Breakfast: Drizzled oatmeal with apple slices, cinnamon, and chia seeds

Lunch: The Buddha bowl of quinoa and chickpeas, tahini dressing.

Dinner: Cornbread with vegan chili.

Day 9:

Breakfast: Greek yogurt, whole grain waffles, and mixed berries

Lunch: Balsamic-glazed caprese salad, whole grain crackers.

Dinner: turkey meatballs on a bed of spaghetti squash cooked in marinara sauce.

Day 10:

Breakfast: Sausage burrito breakfast avocado and egg.

Lunch: Feta-strawberries spinach salad with walnuts.

Dinner: Broccoli, brown rice and teriyaki tofu stir-fry

Keep on consuming of a balanced diet with variety.

Day 11:

Breakfast: Whole grain French toast with fresh berries and honey drizzled over it.

Lunch: Brown rice and vegetables stir-fried with chickpeas

Dinner: quinoa, steamed broccoli, and baked cod with a lemon-herb crust.

Day 12:

Greek yogurt parfait with granola and almond slices for breakfast

Lunch would be a balsamic vinaigrette-topped spinach and mushroom salad.

Supper is vegan enchiladas with sweet potatoes and black beans.

Day 13:

Tofu scrambled with spinach, cherry tomatoes, and turmeric for breakfast

Lunch would be a side of healthy grain bread and lentil and kale soup.

Dinner is sautéed green beans, quinoa, and grilled chicken breast with mango-avocado salsa.

Day 14:

Chia Seed Pudding with sliced peaches and a dash of cinnamon for breakfast

Lunch is a salad of roasted vegetables and quinoa dressed with tahini and lemon juice.

The supper will be a mixed green salad and baked eggplant parmesan.

Day 15:

Cream cheese smoked salmon, and capers on a whole-grain bagel for breakfast

Lunch consists of grilled chicken breast, spinach, and strawberry salad dressed with balsamic vinaigrette.

Dinner is jasmine rice and vegan Thai red curry with tofu.

Day 16:

Omelets with avocado tomato and feta cheese for breakfast

Lunch would be a salad of black beans and corn dressed with lime-cilantro.

Dinner is sautéed spinach, sweet potato wedges, and grilled steak with chimichurri sauce.

Day 17:

Oatmeal with sliced bananas and almond butter for breakfast

Quinoa and Chickpea Stuffed Acorn Squash for lunch

Dinner is quinoa stuffed bell peppers topped with a tomato-basil sauce made vegan.

Day 18:

Mixed berry and granola Greek yogurt smoothie bowl for breakfast

Lunch would be a salad of spinach and lentils dressed with lemon tahini.

Dinner includes steamed asparagus, wild rice, and grilled swordfish marinated in a citrus-herb sauce.

Day 19:

Scrambled eggs with a side of whole grain pancakes topped with maple syrup for breakfast

Lunch would be a balsamic-glazed caprese quinoa salad.

The supper is basmati rice and a vegan curry with chickpeas and vegetables.

Day 20:

Whole grain toast with avocado and egg for breakfast.

Lunch would be pasta with spinach walnut pesto and cherry tomatoes.

Dinner consists of roasted Brussels sprouts, quinoa, and baked halibut in a lemon-dill sauce.

Maintain your commitment to a diversified and well-balanced diet plan. Always remember to stay hydrated throughout the day and to indulge in a variety of nutrient-dense foods. As usual, seek individualized advice from a medical practitioner or qualified nutritionist, particularly if you have certain dietary requirements or health issues.

Remain dedicated to your path to a more vibrant, healthier version of yourself!

CHAPTER 12

The Journey Ahead

When you finish reading this thorough guide on the significant connection between nutrition and health, you should take some time to think back on what you've learned and plan your next steps. The transition to a more conscientious and health-conscious eating style is a thrilling and revolutionary one. In this last chapter, we'll review the most important lessons learned and offer helpful advice to encourage you to keep moving forward in the direction of a better, more conscious relationship with food.

Key Takeaways:

1. Diet Affects All Elements of Health: We've looked at how diet impacts not only your weight but also your vitality, mental health, risk of chronic diseases, and general well-being. Seeing how much your diet affects your health is the first step towards changing for the better.

2. Integral Variety and Equilibrium: To ensure your body gets all the nutrients it needs, you must eat a varied and well-balanced diet rich in

whole grains, lean meats, fruits, vegetables, and healthy fats. To make sure you're getting the right vitamins and minerals, try to vary up your meals.

3. Density of Nutrients Important: The mainstay of your diet should be foods that are high in nutrients compared to calories or those that are nutrient-dense. Leafy greens, berries, almonds, and lean meats are some of these foods. Making nutrient-dense food selections a priority will guarantee you receive the greatest health benefits for your money.

4. Intentional Consumption: Savoring your food, observing hunger cues, and putting away distractions during meals are all part of eating mindfully. By doing this, you can improve your appreciation of food, avoid overindulging, and make healthier decisions.

5. Water is Essential: Maintaining adequate hydration is essential for general health. Water is involved in several processes, including temperature regulation, nutrition absorption, and digestion. Make water your go-to beverage and keep in mind that sometimes hunger and thirst are the same thing.

6. Cooking at Home: You have more control over what ingredients go into your food when you cook at home. It enables you to select high-

quality products, manage portion sizes, and try out new recipes that support your health objectives.

7. Health-Boosting Dietary Practices: Dietary practices that have demonstrated beneficial effects on health include plant-based diets, the Mediterranean diet, and intermittent fasting. Look into these patterns to see which one best fits your tastes and way of life.

8. Tranquility: You have particular dietary demands. When choosing what to eat, take your age, level of activity, and any underlying medical concerns into account. You can tailor your diet for best health by speaking with a medical expert or certified dietitian.

9. Steer clear of processed foods: Foods that have undergone extensive processing frequently include trans fats, added sugars, and harmful ingredients. Reducing the amount of these foods in your diet can improve your overall health and well-being.

10. Healthy Eating: Food preparation, handling, and storage practices can affect your health. It is imperative to comply with food safety regulations to avert foodborne infections.

The Path Forward:

You've only just begun your journey toward eating in a healthier, more mindful way—it doesn't end on the last page of this guide. The following useful actions can assist you in carrying on with this journey:

1. Make definite goals: Establish measurable objectives for your nutrition and overall well-being. Whether your goal is to lose weight, gain more energy, or improve your general well-being, setting specific goals will help you stay motivated.

2. Arrange and Get Ready: Make nutritious snack preparations in advance to keep on hand along with your meal plans. This lessens the likelihood that you will choose unhealthy items out of hunger or distraction.

3. Try Out Novel Recipes: Keep investigating and trying out different recipes. Eating healthily can be exciting and fun when you try new foods and cooking methods.

4. Remain Informed: Keep abreast of current nutritional studies and trends. Being knowledgeable about nutrition will help you make wise decisions because the field is always changing.

5. Seek Support: Talk to people about your experience, get in touch with a trained dietician, or join a support group. It may be simpler to keep on course if you have a support network.

6. Make Mindful Food Choices: Maintain your mindful eating routine. Take note of your body's signals of hunger and fullness, and enjoy the tastes and textures of your food.

7. Get Regular Exercise: To get the most health benefits, combine regular exercise with a nutritious diet. Engaging in physical exercise promotes not just physical health but also emotional wellness.

8. Follow Up on Progress To measure your progress toward your goals, keep a food journal or use a nutrition tracking app. This might support your accountability.

9. Treat Yourself with Kindness: Keep in mind that no one has a flawless diet. It's acceptable to indulge occasionally and to not punish yourself for doing so. Moderation and balance are crucial.

10. Share Your Knowledge: Tell them what you know. Everyone will benefit from a supportive environment that you may establish by inviting friends and family to travel with you.

In conclusion, adopting a more attentive and healthful eating style is a continuous process. It's an educational, transformative, and self-discovery trip. You may significantly improve your health and well-being by implementing the knowledge and insights you've received from this guide in your day-to-day activities. Keep in mind that minor adjustments made consistently might have major effects. I hope you enjoy every bit of this adventure and find plenty of satisfying, nourishing, and tasty experiences along the way. Cheers to being in better health!